CHINESE HERBAL MEDICINE FOR SENIORS POCKET BIBLE

Harnessing The Wisdom Of Traditional Chinese Medicine For Optimal Senior Health

Jones Anderson

Table of contents

INTRODUCTION

A pillar of traditional Chinese medicine (TCM), Chinese herbal medicine has a long and illustrious history that dates back more than two millennia. Its origins can be discovered in ancient China, where a complex system of healing was established based on collected knowledge of medicinal plants and empirical findings.

Early History: The Inception of Chinese Herbal Medicines

Chinese herbal medicine has been documented since the Eastern Han Dynasty (25-220 AD), when important texts such as The Divine Farmer's Materia Medica (Shen Nong Ben Cao Jing) were published. This thorough compilation laid the foundation for future developments and offered practitioners a useful resource by outlining the therapeutic qualities of more than 365 plants.

Refinement and Maturation: A Knowledge Tapestry

Chinese herbal medicine developed over the ages by

incorporating the knowledge of succeeding healing generations. During the Tang Dynasty (618-907 AD), notable advancements were made, one of which being the publication of Li Shizhen's Ben Cao Gang Mu (Compendium of Materia Medica) in 1593. This enormous work established the theoretical foundation of Chinese herbal medicine by carefully classifying and describing over 1,800 therapeutic ingredients.

Adaptation and Integration: Living in Balance with Nature

Chinese herbal medicine, which emphasizes the connection between people and environment, has traditionally been closely associated with the Chinese way of thinking. A key component of TCM is the idea of yin-yang, or the balance of opposing energies, which directs the choice and use of herbal treatments. Herbalists can customise remedies to suit each patient's unique constitution and imbalances by classifying herbs according to their attributes, which include temperature, taste, and meridian affinity.

A Lasting Legacy: A Link to Contemporary Medicine

Chinese herbal medicine continues to be an essential part of healthcare both in China and globally, even with the development of Western medicine. In the field of complementary and alternative medicine, it is well-respected because to its lengthy history and demonstrated effectiveness. The mechanisms of action of herbal treatments are still being studied by researchers today, helping to close the knowledge gap between conventional wisdom and contemporary scientific understanding.

A Look Towards the Future: Upholding Customs, Embracing Innovation

Chinese herbal medicine has both potential and problems as it makes its way through the twenty-first century. It is crucial to embrace the advances of modern science while preserving the integrity of traditional practices. The maintenance of Chinese herbal medicine's efficacy and relevance in the future depends on ongoing study, standardization of herbal formulations, and cooperation between contemporary researchers and traditional practitioners.

The principles of Chinese herbal medicine are founded on a holistic understanding of the body and its relationship to the natural world. These principles emphasize balance, harmony, and the interconnectedness of all things.

1. Yin and Yang

One of the most fundamental concepts in Chinese medicine is the balance of yin and yang. Yin is associated with coolness, darkness, and femininity, while yang is associated with warmth, light, and masculinity. These two forces are constantly interacting and must be in balance for health to be maintained. Herbal remedies are classified according to their yin and yang properties and are used to restore balance to the body.

2. Qi

Qi is the vital energy that flows through the body and nourishes all living things. It is responsible for the proper functioning of the organs and systems of the body. When Qi is blocked or deficient, illness can occur. Chinese herbal medicine aims to regulate Qi flow and restore balance to the body.

3. The Five Elements

The five elements – wood, fire, earth, metal, and water – are another important concept in Chinese medicine. Each element is associated with certain organs, emotions, and physical characteristics. Herbal remedies are also classified according to their elemental properties and are used to address imbalances in the body.

4. Meridian Channels

Meridian channels are the pathways through which Qi flows throughout the body. They are connected to the organs and tissues and play a vital role in maintaining health. Herbal remedies are often used to unblock meridian channels and promote the smooth flow of Qi.

5. Patterns of Dissonance

Chinese herbal medicine practitioners diagnose illness by identifying patterns of dissonance, which are imbalances in the body's energy system. These patterns are based on a combination of symptoms, signs, and diagnostic techniques such as tongue and pulse diagnosis. Herbal remedies are selected based on the specific pattern of dissonance in order to address the root cause of the illness.

6. Individualized Treatment

Chinese herbal medicine is highly individualized and takes into account the unique constitution and needs of each patient. Herbal formulas are often complex and may contain multiple herbs with different properties. The dosage and administration of herbal remedies are also tailored to the individual patient.

7. Holistic Approach

Chinese herbal medicine is part of a larger system of traditional Chinese medicine (TCM), which also includes acupuncture, massage, and dietary therapy. TCM practitioners treat the whole person, not just the symptoms of illness. They aim to restore balance and harmony to the body, mind, and spirit.

IDENTIFYING AND ASSESSING CHINESE HERBAL MEDICINE FOR SENIORS

A cautious and individualized approach is necessary when identifying and evaluating herbal medicines for seniors, taking into account their particular needs, medical problems, and any drug interactions. This is a thorough guide on choosing suitable herbal medicines for elderly people:

1. Speak with a Qualified Medical Expert: It's important to consult your healthcare physician before starting any herbal medicine program. They are able to determine any possible contraindications, evaluate your specific needs, and make sure that herbal therapies work in tandem with your current treatment regimen.

2. Take Into Account Any Underlying Medical Conditions: Seniors frequently have several medical issues that need to be continuously managed. Selecting herbal medicines that won't worsen pre-existing health conditions or interfere with prescription drugs is crucial.

3. Comprehend Drug-Herb Interactions: Numerous herbal therapies have the potential to negatively interact with pharmaceutical medications. Seniors are especially susceptible to these interactions since they frequently take many drugs. To find out whether there are any possible interactions, speak with your healthcare provider.

4. Select Reputable Sources: Invest in herbal treatments from reliable vendors who follow quality assurance guidelines. Steer clear of unreliable suppliers or unlicensed internet sellers while purchasing herbs.

5. Start with Low Doses: As with any herbal therapy, start with low doses and work your way up to a safe level. Keep a watchful eye on your reaction and speak with your doctor if you feel any negative effects.

6. Exercise Consistency and Patience: The effects of herbal therapies may take time to become apparent. To get the best effects, use consistently.

7. Maintain Open Communication: Share any herbal remedies you use with your healthcare physician. Maintaining coordination and safety of your whole treatment plan is ensured by regular contact.

COMMON CHINESE HERBAL MEDICINES FOR SENIORS

Herbs for enhancing energy and vitality

Seniors can increase their vitality and energy levels with a variety of common Chinese herbal medications. Among the most widely used herbs are:

Ginseng: For decades, ginseng has been utilized as a popular herbal medicine to enhance energy levels, cognitive function, and general wellness. It is believed to function by boosting blood flow to the brain and activating the central nervous system.

Reishi Mushrooms: Another adaptogenic plant with a reputation for raising vitality and lowering stress is reishi mushroom. It is also believed to have immune-stimulating and anti-inflammatory qualities.

The Cordyceps: A fungus called cordyceps has long been used to boost energy and enhance sports performance. It is believed to function via lowering tiredness and improving oxygen uptake.

*Astragalus: Herbs like astragalus are frequently used to boost immunity and enhance general health. It is also believed to possess antioxidant and anti-inflammatory qualities.

Berries goji: One kind of fruit that is high in antioxidants and other minerals is goji berry. They are believed to enhance general health, energy levels, and cognitive performance.

There are other ways to consume these herbs, such as tinctures, teas, and capsules. Before using any herbal medicines, it's crucial to see a doctor because they may interfere with some prescriptions.

Apart from consuming herbal treatments, elderly individuals can engage in several additional activities to enhance their energy levels, including:

Eating a nutritious diet: The body can obtain the nutrients it needs to make energy from a diet rich in fruits, vegetables, and whole grains.

Exercising on a regular basis: Regular exercise helps enhance muscle strength, endurance, and cardiovascular health.

Getting adequate sleep: The average adult needs seven to eight hours of sleep every night. Both energy levels and cognitive performance can be enhanced by getting enough sleep.

Managing stress: Fatigue and poor energy are two factors that can be caused by stress. It can be beneficial to find stress-reduction techniques that are healthy, like yoga or meditation.

Seniors can increase their vitality and energy levels and live healthier lives by adopting good lifestyle choices and using herbal medicines under a doctor's supervision.

HERBS FOR IMPROVING SLEEP AND REDUCING STRESS

Here are some herbs that may help improve sleep and reduce stress:

Valerian root: Valerian root is a popular herb that has been used for centuries to treat insomnia and anxiety. It is thought to work by increasing levels of GABA, a neurotransmitter that has calming effects.

Chamomile: Chamomile is a member of the daisy family that has been used for centuries to promote relaxation and sleep. It is thought to work by binding to benzodiazepine receptors in the brain, which are also targeted by anti-anxiety medications.

Lavender: Lavender is a flowering plant that is known for its calming scent. It is thought to work by activating the parasympathetic nervous system, which is responsible for the "rest and digest" response.

Passionflower: Passionflower is a vine that is native to the Americas. It is thought to work by increasing levels of GABA and inhibiting the breakdown of acetylcholine, a neurotransmitter that is involved in memory and learning.

Ashwagandha: Ashwagandha is an herb that has been used in traditional Indian medicine for centuries to treat anxiety and stress. It is thought to work by reducing levels of cortisol, the stress hormone.

L-theanine: L-theanine is an amino acid that is found in green tea. It is thought to work by increasing levels of GABA and dopamine, neurotransmitters that have calming and mood-boosting effects.
[Image of L-theanine amino acid]

Melatonin: Melatonin is a hormone that helps to regulate sleep. It is available as a dietary supplement and is sometimes used to treat insomnia.
[Image of Melatonin hormone]

It is important to note that these herbs are not a substitute for a healthy lifestyle. Getting regular exercise, eating a healthy diet, and managing stress are all important for improving sleep quality. Additionally, some herbs can interact with medications, so it is important to talk to a healthcare professional before taking any new supplements.

HERBS FOR SUPPORTING CARDIOVASCULAR HEALTH

Several herbs have been traditionally used to support cardiovascular health. These herbs may help to improve heart function, reduce blood pressure, and lower cholesterol levels. However, it is important to note that there is limited scientific evidence to support the use of most of these herbs. Additionally, some herbs may interact with medications, so it is important to talk to your doctor before taking them.

Some herbs that are commonly used to support cardiovascular health include:

Hawthorn berry (Crataegus monogyna): Hawthorn berry is a shrub that has been used for centuries to treat heart disease. It is thought to work by improving blood flow to the heart and by strengthening the heart muscle.

Garlic (Allium sativum): Garlic is a vegetable that has been shown to lower cholesterol levels and reduce blood pressure. It is also thought to have anti-inflammatory and antioxidant properties.

Ginger (Zingiber officinale): Ginger is a spice that has been shown to improve blood circulation and reduce blood pressure. It is also thought to have anti-inflammatory and antioxidant properties.

Turmeric (Curcuma longa): Turmeric is a spice that has been shown to lower cholesterol levels and reduce inflammation. It is also thought to have antioxidant and anti-cancer properties.

Omega-3 fatty acids: Omega-3 fatty acids are found in fatty fish, such as salmon, mackerel, and sardines. They are thought to reduce the risk of heart disease by lowering triglycerides and blood pressure.

It is important to note that these herbs are not a substitute for a healthy diet and lifestyle. Eating a healthy diet, exercising regularly, and maintaining a healthy weight are the best ways to reduce your risk of heart disease. If you are considering taking herbs to support your cardiovascular health, it is important to talk to your doctor first.

Here are some additional tips for supporting cardiovascular health:

- Eat a healthy diet that is low in saturated fat, cholesterol, and salt.
- Exercise regularly.
- Maintain a healthy weight.
- Quit smoking.
- Manage stress levels.
- Limit alcohol consumption.

By following these tips, you can help to reduce your risk of heart disease and improve your overall cardiovascular health.

HERBS FOR ENHANCING COGNITIVE FUNCTION AND MEMORY

Traditional Chinese medicine (TCM) has a long history of using herbs to support cognitive function and memory. While more research is needed to confirm the effectiveness of these herbs, some promising candidates include:

Ginkgo biloba (ginkgo): Ginkgo biloba is a tree that has been used for centuries in TCM to improve blood circulation and cognitive function. Some studies suggest that ginkgo biloba may improve memory, attention, and overall cognitive function in people with mild cognitive impairment or early dementia.

Panax ginseng (ginseng): Ginseng is a plant that has been used for centuries in TCM to improve energy levels, mental clarity, and overall health. Some studies suggest that ginseng may improve cognitive function, including memory and attention, in healthy adults and people with mild cognitive impairment.

Cordyceps militaris (cordyceps): Cordyceps is a fungus that has been used for centuries in TCM to improve athletic performance and immune function. Some studies suggest that cordyceps may also improve cognitive function, including memory and learning, in healthy adults and older adults.

Astragalus membranaceus (astragalus): Astragalus is a plant that has been used for centuries in TCM to improve immune function and overall health. Some studies suggest that astragalus may also improve cognitive function, including memory and learning, in healthy adults and older adults.

Rhodiola rosea (rhodiola): Rhodiola is a plant that has been used for centuries in TCM to improve mental clarity, energy levels, and stress resistance. Some studies suggest that rhodiola may also improve cognitive function, including memory and attention, in healthy adults and people with mild cognitive impairment.

It is important to note that these herbs are not a substitute for a healthy lifestyle. Eating a healthy diet, exercising regularly, and getting enough sleep are the best ways to promote cognitive health. If you are considering taking herbs to support your cognitive function, it is important to talk to your doctor first.

Here are some additional tips for enhancing cognitive function and memory:

- Eat a healthy diet that is rich in fruits, vegetables, and whole grains.
- Exercise regularly.
- Get enough sleep.
- Manage stress levels.
- Engage in mentally stimulating activities, such as reading, puzzles, and learning new things.
- Stay socially connected.

By following these tips, you can help to keep your mind sharp and protect your cognitive health.

HERBS FOR STRENGTHENING THE IMMUNE SYSTEM

Traditional Chinese medicine (TCM) has a long history of using herbs to support and strengthen the immune system. While more research is needed to fully understand the mechanisms of action of these herbs, there is growing evidence to suggest that they may offer some benefits for immune health.

Here are some of the most commonly used Chinese herbs for the strengthening of the immune system:

Astragalus root (Huang qi): Astragalus is a well-known adaptogen, a substance that helps the body adapt to stress and maintain homeostasis. It is thought to boost the immune system by increasing the production of white blood cells and enhancing their activity.

Siler root (Du huo): Siler root is another adaptogen that is traditionally used to treat respiratory infections and strengthen the immune system. It is thought to work by stimulating the production of interferon, a protein that helps fight viruses.

Bai-zhu atractylodes rhizome (Bai zhu): Bai-zhu is a bitter herb that is traditionally used to tonify the spleen and stomach. It is also thought to have immune-boosting properties, as it is believed to increase the production of antibodies.

Ganoderma lucidum (Lingzhi): Ganoderma lucidum is a type of mushroom that is highly prized in TCM for its immune-boosting properties. It is thought to work by stimulating the production of white blood cells and macrophages, which are immune cells that help fight infection.

Cordyceps sinensis (Dong chong xia cao): Cordyceps sinensis is a parasitic fungus that is traditionally used to improve respiratory health and strengthen the immune system. It is thought to work by stimulating the production of natural killer cells, which are immune cells that help fight cancer and other infections.

It is important to note that these herbs should not be taken as a substitute for a healthy diet and lifestyle. Eating a balanced diet, getting enough sleep, and managing stress are all important for maintaining a healthy immune system.

If you are considering using Chinese herbs to strengthen your immune system, it is important to talk to a qualified herbalist or healthcare provider. They can help you choose the right herbs for your individual needs and ensure that you are taking them safely and effectively.

HERBS FOR MANAGING CHRONIC PAIN AND INFLAMMATION

Several herbs have been traditionally used to manage chronic pain and inflammation. While more research is needed to confirm the effectiveness of these herbs, some of the most promising options include:

1. Turmeric: Turmeric contains curcumin, a compound with potent anti-inflammatory properties. Studies have shown that curcumin can be as effective as ibuprofen in reducing pain and inflammation in people with osteoarthritis.

2. Ginger: Ginger has been used for centuries to relieve pain and inflammation. It contains gingerols, compounds that have anti-inflammatory and pain-relieving effects. Ginger may be particularly effective in reducing pain from muscle soreness and arthritis.

3. Boswellia: Boswellia is a tree native to India and the Middle

East. Its resin contains boswellic acids, which have anti-inflammatory properties. Studies have shown that boswellia can be effective in reducing pain and inflammation in people with osteoarthritis.

4. Devil's claw: Devil's claw is a vine native to Africa. Its roots contain harpagoside, a compound with anti-inflammatory and pain-relieving effects. Studies have shown that devil's claw can be effective in reducing pain in people with osteoarthritis.

5. White willow bark: White willow bark contains salicin, a compound that is similar to aspirin. Salicin has anti-inflammatory and pain-relieving properties. White willow bark may be effective in reducing pain in people with osteoarthritis and low back pain.

It is important to note that these herbs may interact with certain medications. If you are taking any medications, talk to your doctor before using any herbs.

Here are some additional tips for using herbs to manage chronic pain and inflammation:

- Start with a low dose and increase gradually as needed.
- Take herbs consistently for several weeks to see results.
- Talk to your doctor before using any herbs, especially if you are pregnant or breastfeeding.
- Be aware of potential side effects.

In addition to using herbs, there are other lifestyle changes that can help manage chronic pain and inflammation, such as:

- Eating a healthy diet
- Exercising regularly
- Losing weight

- Getting enough sleep
- Managing stress

If you are struggling with chronic pain or inflammation, talk to your doctor. They can help you develop a treatment plan that includes both conventional and complementary therapies.

INCORPORATING CHINESE HERBAL MEDICINES INTO SENIOR CARE

SELECTING APPROPRIATE HERBAL MEDICINES FOR SENIORS

Chinese herbal medicines can be a useful tool for controlling chronic illnesses and enhancing general health when included in senior care. However, when choosing herbal medications for elders, care must be taken and a customized strategy must be followed.

Tips for Selecting appropriate herbal remedies for seniors

1. Personal Requirements and Health Condition: Every senior has different health requirements and a different medical background. Before suggesting herbal medicines, a thorough evaluation of their general health situation is necessary, taking into account any pre-existing diseases, drugs, and possible sensitivities.

2. Medication and Handling: Elderly people may have different drug metabolisms and sensitivity levels, therefore dose and administration of herbal medications may need to be adjusted. It's usually best to monitor more frequently and use lower dosages.

3. Possible Relationships: Supplements purchased over-the-counter or prescribed drugs may interfere with herbal remedies. In order to prevent unfavorable interactions, thorough communication with the senior's healthcare providers is essential.

4. Sources and Quality: Make sure that the suppliers of herbal medications are reliable and that they follow stringent quality control guidelines. Steer clear of internet markets and unreliable sources when buying herbal treatments.

Choosing the Right Herbal Remedies for Elderly People

1. Address Particular Circumstances: Select herbal remedies that address the senior's particular medical issues. For example, rehmannia may support renal health, while ginseng may be good for cognitive function.

2. Take Into Account Herbal Formulas: Combining several herbs into a mixture known as a polyherbal formula typically offers a more thorough approach to treating complicated health conditions in the elderly.

3. Ask a Knowledgeable Herbalist: Consult a licensed herbalist with knowledge of providing care for the elderly. They are able to determine the specific needs of the elderly person and suggest suitable herbal medicines.

Additional Points to Consider

1. Gradual Introduction: Under the guidance of a medical professional or herbalist, begin with low dosages and progressively increase them.

2. Regular Monitoring: Keep an eye on how the elder is responding to the herbal medications and adjust as necessary.

3. Patient Education: Inform the elderly patient about the possible advantages, drawbacks, and interactions of the herbal remedies.

4. Holistic Approach: Include herbal remedies in a thorough care regimen that also include dietary changes, frequent exercise, and lifestyle alterations.

Recall that adding Chinese herbal remedies to senior care needs to be done so carefully, individually, and under the supervision of licensed medical specialists.

DOSING AND ADMINISTRATION OF CHINESE HERBAL MEDICINES

Dosing and administration of Chinese herbal medicines (CHMs) is a complex and nuanced process that requires careful consideration of various factors, including the patient's age, constitution, diagnosis, and response to treatment. While there are general guidelines for dosing, individualization is crucial to ensure optimal efficacy and safety.

General Dosing Guidelines

CHMs are typically administered in oral liquid form, known as decoctions, which are prepared by boiling herbs in water for a specified period. The dosage of the decoction is usually expressed in grams of herbs per day or per dose. For adults, the average daily dosage of a single herb ranges from 3 to 15 grams, while the average dosage of a polyherbal formula ranges from 15 to 30 grams.

Factors Influencing Dosing

Several factors influence the dosing of CHMs, including:

Age: Children and elderly patients may require lower doses due to their altered pharmacokinetics and sensitivities.

Constitution: Individuals with weaker constitutions may require lower doses than those with stronger constitutions.

Diagnosis: The severity of the disease and the patient's overall health status also influence the dosage.

Response to Treatment: The patient's response to treatment should be closely monitored, and dosage adjustments made as needed.

Administration Methods

CHMs can be administered in various ways, including:

Decoctions: The most common method, decoctions are prepared by boiling herbs in water and then straining the liquid. The decoction can be taken warm or cold, typically divided into two or three doses per day.

Pills: Pills are convenient and easy to administer, often prescribed for long-term treatment. They are prepared by concentrating herbal extracts into a solid form.

Powders: Herbal powders are typically mixed with water or honey before consumption. They are often used for acute conditions or to supplement other forms of CHM administration.

Topical Applications: CHMs can also be applied externally, such as in ointments, plasters, or compresses, for localized pain, inflammation, or skin conditions.

Safety Considerations

CHMs, like any medication, can have potential side effects or interactions with other medications. It is crucial to inform the healthcare provider about all medications, supplements, and herbal remedies being taken to avoid potential adverse interactions.

Consulting a Qualified Practitioner

Due to the complexity of dosing and administration, consulting a qualified practitioner of Chinese herbal medicine is essential. They can assess the patient's individual needs, formulate appropriate dosages, and monitor the patient's response to treatment, ensuring optimal efficacy and safety.

INTEGRATING CHINESE HERBAL MEDICINES WITH WESTERN MEDICINE

Combining Chinese herbal medicine (CHM) with Western medicine can be an effective approach to treating a variety of health conditions. However, it is important to consult with a qualified healthcare professional before using any herbal medicines, as they can interact with Western medications.

Here are some general guidelines for using CHM alongside Western medicine:

Talk to your doctor. It is important to talk to your doctor before using any herbal medicines, as they can interact with Western medications. Your doctor can help you determine if CHM is right for you and can monitor your progress while you are taking it.

Start with a low dose. When you first start taking CHM, it is important to start with a low dose and gradually increase it as needed. This will help to reduce the risk of side effects.

Be patient. It may take several weeks or even months to see the full benefits of CHM. Be patient and continue taking your medication as directed by your healthcare provider.

Be aware of potential side effects. Some herbal medicines can cause side effects, such as stomach upset, headache, or dizziness. If you experience any side effects, talk to your doctor or pharmacist.

Here are some specific examples of how CHM can be used alongside Western medicine:

Pain management. CHM can be used to relieve pain from a variety of conditions, such as arthritis, cancer, and low back pain.

Mental health conditions. CHM can be used to treat a variety of mental health conditions, such as anxiety, depression, and insomnia.

Chronic diseases. CHM can be used to treat chronic diseases, such as diabetes, heart disease, and high blood pressure.

It is important to note that CHM is not a cure-all and should not be used to replace Western medicine. However, it can be a valuable tool for managing chronic conditions and improving overall health and well-being.

Here are some additional tips for using CHM alongside Western medicine:

Choose a qualified practitioner. When choosing a

practitioner of CHM, it is important to choose someone who is qualified and experienced. You can ask your doctor for a referral or search online for a practitioner in your area.

Be honest with your practitioner. Be honest with your practitioner about all of your medical conditions, the medications you are taking, and any herbal remedies you are using. This will help your practitioner to create a treatment plan that is safe and effective for you.

Keep a record of your progress. Keep a record of your progress while you are taking CHM. This will help you to track your symptoms and see if the treatment is working for you.

By following these guidelines, you can safely and effectively use CHM alongside Western medicine to improve your health and well-being.

Remember, Chinese herbal medicines are not a substitute for Western medical care, but rather a complementary therapy that can be used alongside conventional treatments. If you are considering using Chinese herbal medicines, it is important to consult with a qualified healthcare professional to discuss your individual needs and treatment options.

SPECIAL CONSIDERATIONS FOR SENIORS USING CHINESE HERBAL MEDICINES

HERBAL REMEDIES FOR SENIORS WITH COEXISTING CONDITIONS

There are many herbs that are potentially safe for seniors with coexisting conditions. However, it is important to talk to a doctor before starting any new herbal regimen, as some herbs can interact with medications or have other side effects.

Some herbs that are generally considered safe for seniors include:

Chamomile: Chamomile is a calming herb that can be used to treat anxiety, insomnia, and digestive problems. It is available in tea form, capsules, and extracts.

Elderberry: Elderberry is a fruit that has been shown to boost the immune system and fight off infections. It is available in syrup, capsules, and gummies.

Ginger: Ginger is a spice that can help with nausea, vomiting, and indigestion. It is available in fresh, dried, and powdered form.

Ginseng: Ginseng is an adaptogen that can help improve energy levels and reduce stress. It is available in capsules, powders, and teas.

Peppermint: Peppermint is an herb that can help with digestive problems, headaches, and muscle pain. It is available in tea form, capsules, and oil.

Turmeric: Turmeric is a spice that has anti-inflammatory properties and may help with arthritis and other chronic conditions. It is available in capsules, powders, and curcumin extracts.

It is important to note that this is not an exhaustive list, and there are many other herbs that may be safe for seniors. However, it is always best to talk to a doctor before starting any new herbal regimen.

Here are some additional tips for using herbs safely:

- Start with a low dose and increase gradually as needed.

- Take herbs with food to help reduce the risk of stomach upset.
- Be aware of potential interactions with medications.
- Stop using herbs if you experience any side effects.

If you are a senior with coexisting conditions, it is important to work with a healthcare team to find a safe and effective herbal regimen for you.

CONCLUSION

Chinese herbal medicine (CHM) has been used for millennia to treat a variety of illnesses, and its potential advantages in the treatment of elderly patients are becoming more widely acknowledged. CHM is a comprehensive approach to health that aims to bring the body back into harmony and balance. It can be used to treat a range of common health issues that older persons face, including:

Control of pain: Numerous pain conditions, including neuropathic, spinal, and arthritic pain, can be treated with CHM. Research has indicated that CHM may have fewer adverse effects and, in certain situations, be just as effective as traditional painkillers.

The state of your heart: By lowering blood pressure, cholesterol, and enhancing circulation, CHM can help to enhance cardiovascular health. Research has demonstrated the potential benefits of CHM in both treating and preventing cardiac disease.

Mental process: CHM can help elderly persons with their memory and cognitive function. Research has demonstrated that CHM can lessen inflammation and increase blood flow to the brain, both of which can assist to stave off cognitive loss.

Disorders of sleep: Insomnia and other sleep disorders can be treated with CHM. Research has indicated that CHM may be useful in enhancing the length and quality of sleep.

General state of health: By raising mood, lowering stress, and increasing energy, CHM can help older persons' general well-being. Research has indicated that CHM can significantly enhance elderly persons' quality of life.

When used properly, CHM is usually thought to be safe for older persons. But before using any herbal medicines, it's crucial to speak with a trained professional because some herbs have contraindications or may combine with other prescriptions.

Here are a few more advantages of CHM in senior care:

Individualised approach: When creating a treatment plan, CHM professionals consider each patient's unique needs and circumstances. Because they frequently have complicated health demands, older folks can benefit greatly from this individualized approach.

Holistic approach: CHM treats the patient as a whole, not simply the illness's symptoms. This all-encompassing strategy can enhance general health and wellbeing.

A few unfavorable effects: When used properly, CHM is usually thought to be safe for older persons. This is so because

CHM herbs are generally well-tolerated natural compounds.

All things considered, CHM can be a useful tool for enhancing older individuals' health and wellbeing. To create a safe and efficient treatment plan, make sure to speak with a skilled practitioner if you're thinking about utilizing CHM.